THE CARNIVORE DIET

A Beginners Guide to Eating Only Meat

WILL PYKOSZ

Second edition
Typeset edited by Elizabeth Rus

CONTENTS

INTRODUCTION

The Carnivore Diet
A beginners guide to eating only meat

I am writing this book because I have had great results on the carnivore diet. Like many thousands of others, I want to share those results.

I am not a doctor or in the medical profession, so you should not consider anything in this book as medical advice. You should always consult your doctor (if you still do that) before radically changing your diet. My story is just anecdotal until many more studies come out, and they are. Every day, more doctors are coming to understand how they have been steering us wrong for a long time. I have nothing against doctors, but most are so entrenched in the system that they don't have time to keep up with the newer studies. "A pill for every ill" supports the pharmaceutical companies and does not do much, if anything at all, to fix the underlying health problem.

I felt I had to take my health into my own hands, so the journey began. I was 80 pounds overweight and a type 2 Diabetic on the standard medication and feeling like crap.

When the Atkins diet came out, I learned that starches (made from grains and roots) were not good for me. I quit them and healed some.

Then I found the 8-Week Blood Sugar Diet by Dr Michael Mosley. I lost my first 40 pounds, felt great, and went off all medications.

It did not last. I put the weight back on and went back on meds. This diet was not sustainable for me.

Then I came across the Carnivore Diet (after trying several others) a very sustainable diet for me. I lost 50 pounds in a year and kept it off. I am off all meds again, my blood values are normal, and my doctor put in my record that I was no longer a type 2 diabetic. I have no intention of going back.

In the pages that follow, I will tell you how I Carnivore. The diet saved my life. I am now 70 years old, and I hope to live another 30 years

Will

CHAPTER 1:
WHAT IS THE CARNIVORE DIET

Carnivore noun car·ni·vore flesh-*eating animal especially any of an order of flesh-eating mammals*

The carnivore diet is a subset of the Ketogenic diet. The ketogenic diet is carbohydrate-restricted. The fewer carbohydrates you consume, the closer you become to eating like a carnivore.

Most ketogenic diets allow a daily consumption of carbohydrates based on a percentage like ten or twenty percent of daily intake. You eat as close to zero carbs as possible on the carnivore diet. In the carnivore world, there are four basic levels when starting.

1. Ketovore, mostly meat with minimal carbs. Coined by Dr. Ken Berry's wife, Nisha.

2. BBBE. Beef, Bacon, Butter, and Eggs, where beef can be any meat

3. Carnivore, all meat, no carbs, some spices

4. Lyon's Diet. The most restrictive. Mostly red meat but allows ruminant animals, sheep, deer, cows, and any animal with more than one stomach.

CHAPTER 2: WHY CHOOSE THIS DIET

The tribal knowledge of the most physically unfit population on the planet is of no use to me. Unknown

When you decide you are not well, whether it is your weight, a metabolic disorder, or any number of non-communicable diseases, you will go to doctors, and they will most likely put you on pills and refer you to the American diabetes society diet plan or the American Heart Association diet, and tell you that other diets like the Mediterranean diet are how you should eat. This is what happened to me. I am not a doctor or in the medical profession, so my response was my decision and should not be considered medical advice. When listening to my doctor tell me how to eat, I noticed he was not in shape. He was about 60 pounds overweight and clearly did not take his own advice; I told him so and never returned to him. I still had to pay for the visit.

What is healthy eating? When you ask people what that

is, you get many different answers. From going Vegan to buying the best quality food you can buy, but does your health improve? Yes, for a while. Then, you will need to start taking a lot of supplements to get all the nutrients you need (see Dr Chaffee's work below), and you will need to Add fiber, so your intestines work better.

So, what are we to eat? Dr. Ken Berry has coined the term PHD for Proper Human Diet. Looking at the world, we see that all the animals instinctively know what they are supposed to eat except us. And yes, we are an animal on this planet. When you go to the zoo, the signs say, "Don't feed the animals," because they get sick if they eat something not on their natural diet. If 70 to 80 percent of people (depending on who you listen to) in this country alone are overweight or obese, what does this say about our diet, the food pyramid, and the advice our doctors give us?

The cave paintings from 20,000 years ago show hunters with spears hunting animals, not vegetables. The agricultural revolution came about after the end of the last ice age about 12,000 years ago when the large mammals died off, and agriculture became necessary for our survival. When we look at the archaeological record from that time, we find hunter-gatherer villages next to agricultural villages, and we find the beginnings of most of the ills of our culture in the agricultural villages. Bad and crooked teeth, smaller brain size, and famines. A whole book can be written on this subject alone; I will save this for another book. But see Dr. Chaffee's YouTube videos in the meantime. Cited below.

We live in a culture of plenty; mostly, whatever we want

is at arm's reach. We think we work hard and should eat whatever we want because we deserve it; it's our reward. But don't we also deserve good health? Looking around you, most are not healthy; you can choose not to be like them or say that will not be me.

There is not a published diet out there that will kill you in 30 days, not even fasting (under supervision). I did a nine-day fast once and only drank electrolytes. I felt great and only started eating again because it felt weird not to eat.

So, try Carnivore for 30 days, and if you don't think it worked well for you, stop and go back to what you were doing before, but if you feel good, see good results, and are clear-headed, keep going. I'm at 300 days now and have no intention of going back.

CHAPTER 3: HOW TO START

"Good nutrition is always an excellent starting point in regaining health."

— *Steven Magee*

You have decided to try a carnivore diet; there are some things to consider. If you live alone, it will be much easier than if you live with family. Your inner circle of people and friends need to know what you are doing and why and should be onboard and asked not to be enablers. That being said, the willpower ultimately has to come from you. I will proceed as if you live alone, and you will have to adapt to your living situation.

It should be mentioned that you could experience something called the Keto Flu. After a week or two. This happens when your body switches over from burning carbohydrates as fuel to burning fat and producing ketones for fuel. When burning carbohydrates as fuel, it is necessary to refuel often; that is why we eat three times a day and some six times. It takes between one to three weeks when we switch to Carnivore for your body to burn off all its stored glucose and convert to burning fat. This process of switching over can be experienced as flu-like symptoms. They last only a few days, and not all experience this. Also, some can experience lightheadedness and possible dizziness, almost like low blood sugar. Test your sugar to find out. If your blood sugar is low, you may need to consult your doctor and have your meds adjusted. This diet will naturally lower blood sugar. But you may also just be dehydrated. Drink good, clean water and add sugar-free electrolytes (no artificial sweeteners if possible.), and don't forget to eat; most people do not eat enough at first on the carnivore diet.

On the carnivore diet, we eat only meat, so my main man, Dr

Anthony Chaffee, MD, says, "Plants are trying to kill you." This is not with overt intent but in all their defense chemicals. I will link to this video below. It was instrumental in my decision to go Carnivore.

So, if you get rid of all plants, what does that mean? It means you get rid of anything made from plants. This is huge. It means all pasta, grains, cereals, bread, rice, flour, and starch, SUGAR, all root vegetables, fruits, spices, potato chips (chips are the only thing I still miss), snacks, seed oils, and anything that contains the above. Yes, you do have to read labels. Also, dairy (eggs are not dairy; they are just kept by the dairy section for refrigeration) so if you say, I am not going to eat sugar or anything that turns to sugar in my body… you are a carnivore because protein and fat are all that is left.

Dr. Paul Saladino is a Carnivore but has added fruit back into his diet, link below for his reasons and website. So, get rid of all this stuff from your house. It is easier if you have no temptations.

Go to the store and buy meat.

CHAPTER 4: WHAT TO EAT, HOW MUCH, AND WHEN.

I didn't claw my way to the top of the food chain to eat vegetables.

Meat is in, and plants are out; all kinds of meats are okay when starting, and the longer I have been on this diet, the more I am gravitating towards red meat. It just makes me feel better.

- Beef
- Venison
- Lamb
- Goat
- Pork
- Chicken

- Seafood

- Shellfish

And any other meat you like.

The best animals to eat are ruminant animals; these are the ones that have more than one stomach, like beef, lamb, goat, venison, and others.

This is because the additional stomachs can digest the

native plant toxins, so they are not absorbed into the meat of the animals. The single stomach animals like chicken and pork cannot digest the plant toxins and absorb them into their meat, which we then ingest.

Natural plant toxins or phytochemicals are defense chemicals plants use to protect themselves from predators, insects, disease, and being eaten. The common ones we know of are lectins and oxalates, and the debate is still on whether gluten is a toxin. But if we are not eating plants, we are not eating gluten.

Grass-fed vs. grain-fed, Grass-fed meat, by all standards, is better than grain-fed meat, and if you can afford it and it is available in your area, it is a good choice. But don't let the perfect get in the way of the good. The ruminant animals can digest most of the plant toxins in grain-fed animals. When you start, eat what is available and within your budget, and as you progress, become pickier.

What to Drink

I mostly drink water, filtered or distilled. I do this myself at home and avoid plastic bottles when possible. I add electrolytes that I make myself. I will put a link below to how this is done. I still drink coffee and some teas, and though they are made from plants, they don't bother me. I have tried to quit coffee, and I think kicking heroin would be easier.

It is not good to drink alcohol, and though it is an accepted part of society, and I drank for years, it is still a slow poison and full of sugar. And it is very damaging to your liver and health. My best to you if quitting this is also part of your journey.

The actual eating part, how much and how often

I don't stop eating when I'm full. The meal isn't over when I'm full. It's over when I hate myself, Louis C. K.

Do not count calories on a carnivore diet; instead, think about how many pounds to eat in a day; somewhere between one and two pounds a day should be good for most people, but if you spend all day in the gym, it might be more. Eating meat, you are eating fat and protein; About 70 percent of your calories should come from fat and the rest from protein (see Dr. Chaffee et al. below). This seemed excessive to me, and I kept my food to only one pound a day and did not lose weight. When I increased from 1.5 pounds to two pounds, my weight dropped. It seems strange, but it works for me. Some people tell you to stop weighing yourself, some once a week, some every day. I like the feedback every day. This should be what seems alright to you.

To weigh or not to weigh

Depending on who you talk to, they will tell you not to weigh yourself, but maybe once a week or every two weeks, and some will tell you that weighing every day is okay. I like to weigh every day; I like feedback. If I lost, I did well yesterday, and if I gained, I did not so well. Also, when you start, you should take some measurements, waist, hips, etc., because if you stall in weight loss, you could be gaining muscle and losing inches, and this is equally good.

First, eat as much as you want and as many times a day as you are used to. It is essential to get rid of the stored sugar (glucose) in your body so that you can start burning ketones as soon as possible. Once you are in fat-burning mode, you will find that you won't want to eat as often. You will forget to eat; this happens when your body gets the necessary nutrients. You will find you only need to eat once or twice a day. I usually eat once a day, called OMAD (one meal a day), and sometimes I add breakfast. Remember to keep the food weight up, and if you can't eat it all at once, finish it in a few hours. Dr Chaffee (below) says you should stop eating when the food stops tasting good. If it stops tasting good halfway through, put it away for later. If it tastes good and your plate is empty, consider eating more. Throughout the years, I have heard many diet advisors say to listen to your body without telling you what to listen for. Eating until it stops tasting good was the first concrete indicator I heard, along with the results of eating too much or too little fat.

A couple of other considerations. Because this diet contains no plants, it also contains no fiber. The medical profession is now trying to say that fiber is an essential nutrient. The term essential nutrient means you will die if you don't eat it. All our food can be classified into three categories: protein, fat, and carbohydrates. There are essential fats and proteins but no essential carbohydrates (fiber would be a carbohydrate even though it is indigestible). This can easily be shown by looking at the Eskimos (Dr. Chaffee et al.), who lived only on fat and animal protein because plants do not grow there. They did not die off and were perfectly healthy until we introduced them to our diet, then they got all our diseases.

In the 1970s, we were told to stop eating saturated fats, reduce meat consumption, and eat more grains and vegetables. Grains and vegetables bind up our intestines, so we were told more fiber was needed to loosen things up. And the recommendation for more dietary fiber goes up every few years.

All of this is brought up because of the concern that we do not get fiber on a carnivore diet. Remember, the Eskimos ate no fiber. So how is this addressed in the carnivore diet, with fat! If you use the restroom too frequently, you are eating too much fat, and if you seem constipated, you are not using enough fat. After you transition to Carnivore, you will find that not using the restroom more than two to three times a week becomes normal, sometimes less. This is because most of what you eat is completely digested (meat does not rot in your intestines.), so there is much less to pass through.

CHAPTER 5: HOW NOT TO GET BORED OF JUST MEAT

Find joy in the process, not just the outcome. Focus on the journey, not just the destination.

As long as you only eat meat, salt, and water, your body will not get bored; the rest is in your head. When you start adding things back, the trouble begins. First, it's a little spice, then more spice. Next, you have a potato or a salad, and then you are no longer a carnivore. There is a lot of social pressure to keep you eating like the herd, not to mention the pressure you put on yourself to be polite, not offend anyone, and be part of the pack. At first, you will feel like a lone wolf; wait a second, a wolf is a carnivore. There are more of us out there than you think. This diet has many variations, including types of meat, cooking methods, and combinations. I find three types of meat on the plate make a meal look less boring. It also helps to have a friend who is doing this with you. It helps to keep each other on track

I will link below to a short YouTube video by Max German. He does a great job on this topic.

CHAPTER 6: COOKING ON THIS DIET

"Cooking may be as much a means of expression as any of the arts."   *Fannie Farmer*

The cooking techniques on the carnivore diet are much the same among them are:

- Grilling
- Frying
- Smoking
- Baking
- Roasting
- Slow Cooking
- Sous Vide

With a few exceptions, No spices, and very specific oils.

The only thing I use on meat is salt, and I never put it on until after it is cooked. This is a habit I got into when I still used spices; they just seemed to burn and did not taste as well. Many chiefs will argue this point. This would be your preference. Since there are no plants or seed oils, these would be corn, soy, peanut, canola, and Crisco. The best oils/fats to use are Tallow, rendered beef fat. Lard rendered pork fat. Ghee clarified butter. And other saturated fats. Some fruit oils not made from the seed are okay, like extra virgin olive oil and cold-pressed avocado oil.

It's great if you can find a local butcher who can cut your steaks to whatever thickness you like. I usually have them cut to 1.5 inches; this way, they crisp up enough, and I can keep the inside at a medium rare. If they get any thinner, they get overcooked. I suspect this is because my grill won't get hot enough. The butcher also mixes my hamburger to whatever percentage I want. When grilling in the summer, I mix it to 60/40 percent and grill it to medium rare, but this mix is not suitable for frying because too much fat comes out. I have it mixed at 80/20 percent for indoor cooking in the winter months. This works well in the frying pan.

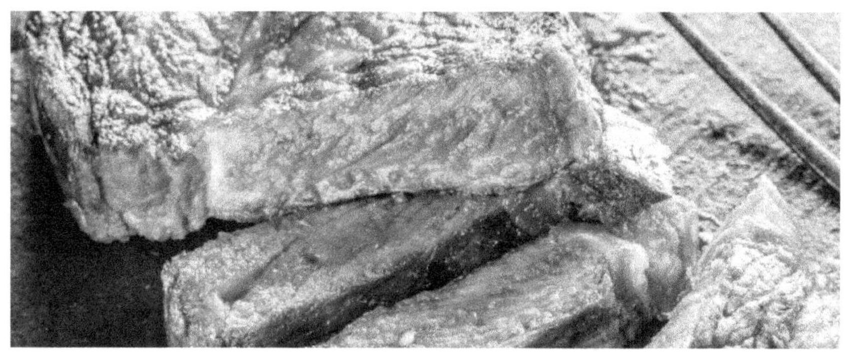

CHAPTER 7: 5
SIMPLE RECIPES

A recipe is a story that ends with a good meal. -Pat Conroy

My favorite is a Ribeye steak

Arguably the most expensive, if not close to it, but if a pound to a pound and a half steak is my total intake for the day it's not bad. I like to dry brine-age my steaks before grilling them. I will provide a link below on how to do this. Lightly salt on all sides and place on a drying rack uncovered in the refrigerator for three to seven days. The flavor is concentrated, and the steaks taste great. The longer they age, less time is needed on the grill. After aging to your preference, they can be frozen. I use a remote thermometer to get the internal temperature to medium rare, and my grill temperature is about 550 degrees. With so many people trying to tell you the perfect way to grill steak, you need to find out what you like. Because this is already salted, you may not need any more salt.

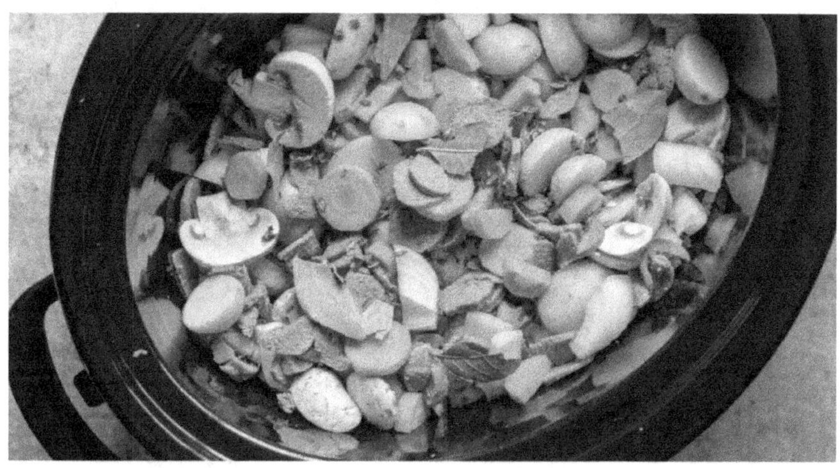

Pork Shoulder in a crockpot

This one is the easiest for me. Just place the shoulder or butt in the crockpot. Fat side up; no added liquid is necessary. I add a little salt, and this is one of the few spices I use a few sprigs of rosemary I cut from a bush in my ward. Set the crockpot to high or low, depending on your time. On high, mine is done in four to five hours.

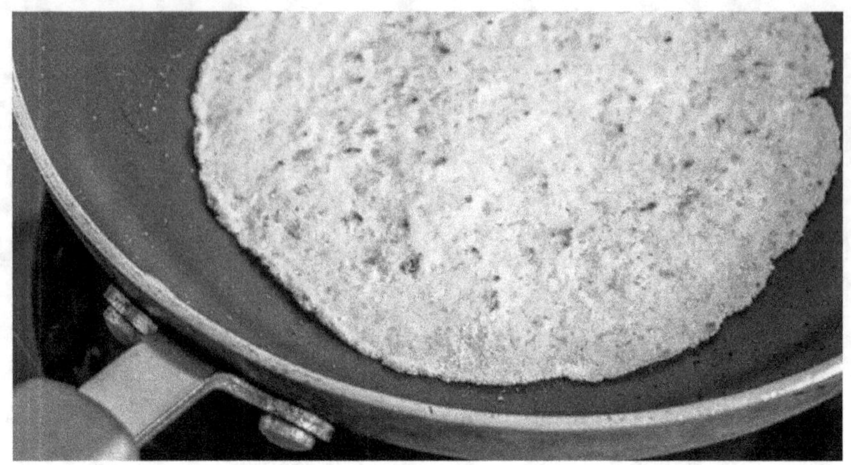

Egg pancakes or Tortillas

Mine are different than the ones you can find on the web; I don't add things to make it look like the pancake you are used to; mine are basically omelets. Eggs with some salt, fried with bacon fat or real butter. Using a pan about the size you want the pancake to be is good. Two eggs in a smaller pan can become stackable, and four eggs in a larger pan can give you the size of a tortilla or burrito; they will need to be cooked a little longer to firm up so they can be rolled or folded. I usually stuff or layer with bacon, a clean sausage (few additives or make your own), chopped leftover steak, chicken, or whatever you have. You can use cheese; the older the cheese is, the harder, the better. I won't usually use cheese because it can stop weight loss. The jury is still out on whether eggs are good for you and how many you should eat. I side with those who say they are good for you and have no quantity issues. I can eat a dozen or more a week and do not have cholesterol issues.

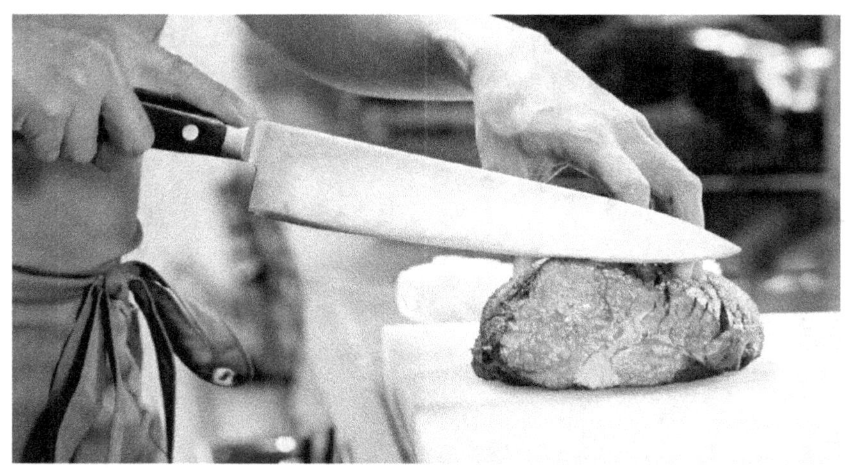

Ribeye Roast

This is one roast that I don't think I have ever found a way to cook that I didn't like. From smoking to slow cooking, my favorite way is in an oven. But I have done it on a grill with little success (still working on it). Set the oven to 500 degrees, and rub the roast with salt. When the oven is at temperature, put the roast in for five minutes a pound or until you get the sear the way you like it. Reduce the heat to 350 degrees and cook for 10 to 15 minutes per pound for medium rare. I always use a temperature probe to get this part right. And as usual, let it rest.

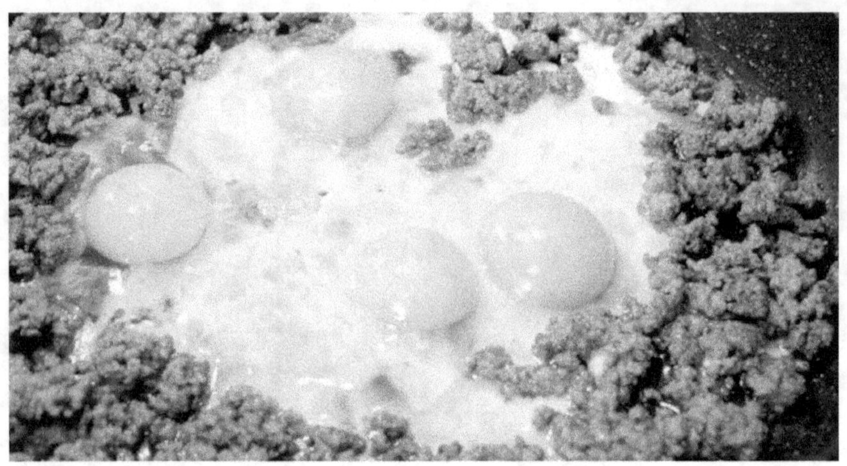

Ground beef and eggs

This is one to have fun with, and it has a lot of variations. In a frying pan, use about a pound of ground beef, chopped steak, or chicken, and add some bacon if you like, and brown. Add eggs four or five and scramble or leave them whole; add a tablespoon of water, cover, reduce heat, and steam until the eggs are cooked how you like them. I like a soft yoke. Add cheese if you like, depending on where you are on the Carnivore diet.

CHAPTER 8: FURTHER EDUCATION

One of the things that keeps me motivated is continuing my education. I rarely skip a day watching a video from one of my subscribed YouTube channels or reading a book on health or the carnivore lifestyle. And it won't take long to realize that unless your doctor is keto-friendly, you can quickly know more about nutrition than your doctor does. I was asking a doctor a few years ago about lab tests and treatment for type 2 diabetes and was told by the doctor; I can't pay attention to that cutting-edge science you are asking about; I have to treat you with the standard of care (the classic way diabetes is treated. A year later, she was the doctor who put in my record that I was no longer diabetic. She wanted to know how I did it, so I told her it was the Mediterranean diet. I did not feel like an argument since she already told me the carnivore diet was unhealthy.

The following are some YouTube channels and books I found helpful. They are not in any specific order. Some are also listed in the reference section below.

Dr. Ken Berry

https://www.youtube.com/@KenDBerryMD

His book: Lies My Doctor Told Me

Dr. Shawn Baker https://www.youtube.com/@ShawnBakerMD

His book The Carnivore Diet

Dr. Anthony Chaffee https://www.youtube.com/@anthonychaffeemd

High Intensity Health https://www.youtube.com/@Highintensityhealth

Max German

https://www.youtube.com/@max.german

Dr. Eric Berg

https://www.youtube.com/@Drberg

Dr. Sten Ekberg

https://www.youtube.com/@drekberg

Thomas Delauer https://www.youtube.com/

@ThomasDeLauerOfficial

Dr. Paul Saladino https://www.youtube.com/@Paulsaladinomd

Low Carb Down Under https://www.youtube.com/@lowcarbdownuunder

Dr. Sean Omara

https://www.youtube.com/@DrSeanOMara

Evil Food Supply https://www.youtube.com/@EvilFoodSupply

Neisha

https://www.youtube.com/@NeishaSalasBerry

Steak and Butter Gal https://www.youtube.com/@SteakandButterGal

Mark Sissions: The Primal Blueprint found on Amazon

These are only some, but it's a good start.

CHAPTER 9: THE BEGINNING

When one door closes, another opens.

Eating Carnivore is not just a diet for me, but now a way of life. And one that I wish I had found 30 years ago. It no longer bothers me when I go to someone's house, and they put a plate of spaghetti in front of me to say I'm sorry, it looks great, but I don't eat that kind of food. It does not go over well sometimes, but mostly it does. There is almost always something in a restaurant you can eat; if not, drink a glass of water or a coffee and be social. That is what you are out for anyway.

I reject the Standard American Diet (SAD diet), and the more people that do, the healthier as a nation we will become.

You can get a lot of flak from Vegans/vegetarians; their belief is almost a religion, and most of it is emotional and not founded in actual studies; there are far more studies on the ketogenic diet than on plant-based diets, and for a vegetarian to be healthy, they need to take a lot of supplements because many nutrients they need can only be found in meats. If you ever get into a discussion with them, it will almost always turn into a shouting match. Even somewhat militant. And I have found that the one that shouts the loudest knows the least. I avoid them whenever possible.

Thank you for buying and reading my book. I believe the Carnivore diet is the PHD (proper human diet), and I hope you come to believe that too.

Thank you,

Will Pykosz

Resources

"Carnivore." Merriam-Webster.com Dictionary, https://www.merriam-webster.com/dictionary/carnivore.

Dr. Ken Berry: https://www.youtube.com/@KenDBerryMD

PHD proper human diet also Dr. Ken Berry

Nisha Berry https://www.youtube.com/@NeishaSalasBerry

Dr Anthony Chaffee MD.

https://www.youtube.com/@anthonychaffee md

Dry-brine aging steaks Dr Anthony Chaffee MD.

https://www.youtube.com/watch?v=yiAOHtV2xrc

Plants are trying to kill you, Dr Anthony Chaffee, MD.
https://www.youtube.com/watch?v=uMahgg9tVUc

DR. Michael Mosley

https://www.amazon.co.uk/8-Week-Blood-Sugar-Diet-reprogramme/dp/1780722400

Dr. Paul Saladino MD https://www.youtube.com/@Paulsaladinomd

Cole Robinson calls the electrolyte recipe snake juice. This guy is a bit crude, so beware https://www.youtube.com/watch?v=1onQ0nxgWFM

Max German How not to get bored

https://www.youtube.com/watch?v=3es5sFeAA1Y